AGE-PROOF

unlock the secrets to a younger, healthier you

ESTHER C. EXCEL

Age-Proof

Table of contents

INTRODUCTION

Welcome to Age Proof: Unlock the Secrets to a Younger, Healthier You

Imagine waking up every morning feeling like you're 25 again - full of energy, vitality, and a zest for life. No more creaky joints, no more brain fog, no more feeling like you're losing your edge. This is the promise of age-proof.

Jane, a vibrant and energetic woman in her early 50s, who seemed to have it all - a successful career, a loving family, and a passion for life. But beneath the surface, Jane was struggling with the telltale signs of aging - fatigue, memory loss, and aching joints. She felt like she was losing herself in the process.

One day, Jane stumbled upon a revolutionary approach to aging - Age Proof. She discovered that aging is not inevitable, and that it's possible to take control of your biological clock and live a younger, healthier life.

In the following pages, we'll take you on a journey to unlock the secrets of Age Proof. You'll discover how to:

- Fuel your body with the right foods and nutrients
- Unlock the power of exercise and movement
- Manage stress and cultivate relaxation
- Build strong social connections
- Stay mentally sharp and focused

Through storytelling, real-life examples, and expert insights, we'll show you how to take control of your aging process and live a younger, healthier life. Join us on this transformative journey, and discover the secrets of Age Proof.,

The Quest for Eternal Youth: A Timeless Pursuit

In the depths of human history, a profound and enduring quest has captivated the imagination of civilizations, philosophers, and scientists alike - the pursuit of eternal youth. This timeless aspiration has driven innovation, discovery, and exploration, as individuals and societies seek to unlock the secrets of a long, healthy, and vibrant life.

Meet Leonardo, a curious and ambitious alchemist from the Renaissance era, who spent his life searching for the Philosopher's Stone - a mythical substance believed to grant eternal life and youth.

Though his quest remained elusive, Leonardo's journey symbolizes the human desire to transcend mortality and defy the constraints of time.

Fast-forward to the present day, when scientists like Dr. Maria, a renowned gerontologist, dedicate their lives to understanding the biology of aging. She's on the cusp of a groundbreaking discovery, one that could potentially reverse the aging process.

Through their stories, we'll explore the fascinating history of the quest for eternal youth, from ancient myths to modern-day breakthroughs. We'll delve into the latest research, expert insights, and innovative strategies for optimizing your health span.

The quest for eternal youth is not just a fantasy; it's a testament to human resilience, curiosity, and the unrelenting desire to push beyond the boundaries of what's possible.

What to Expect from this Book: Unlocking the Secrets to a Younger, Healthier You

As you embark on this journey with Age Proof, you may wonder what secrets lie within its pages. What mysteries will be revealed? What discoveries will be made? And how will your life be transformed by the end of this journey?

Meet Emily, a busy professional in her late 30s, who felt like she was losing her edge. She was tired, stressed, and struggling to keep up with the demands of modern life.

However, after applying the principles outlined in Age Proof, Emily experienced a profound transformation. She regained her energy, clarity, and passion for life.

In the following pages, you'll discover the same secrets that helped Emily unlock a younger, healthier version of herself. You'll learn how to:

- Fuel your body with the right foods and nutrients
- Unlock the power of exercise and movement
- Manage stress and cultivate relaxation
- Build strong social connections
- Stay mentally sharp and focused

Through storytelling, real-life examples, and expert insights, we'll show you how to take control of your aging process and live a longer, healthier, and more fulfilling life. You'll discover:

- The latest scientific breakthroughs in longevity research

- Practical strategies for optimizing your healthspan

- Inspiring stories of people who have successfully applied these principles

By the end of this book, you'll be equipped with the knowledge, tools, and inspiration to unlock a younger, healthier version of yourself. Join us on this transformative journey, and discover the secrets of Age Proof.

PART ONE: UNDERSTANDING AGING

CHAPTER 1: The Biology of Aging: What Happens as We Age

Rachel is a vibrant and energetic woman in her early 40s, who began to notice subtle changes in her body. She felt tired more easily, her skin lost its luster, and her memory wasn't as sharp as it used to be. Rachel wondered, "What's happening to me? Is this what aging feels like?"

As we age, our bodies undergo a series of complex changes that affect our cells, tissues, and organs. It's a natural process, but one that can be influenced by our lifestyle choices.

Let's explore the fascinating biology of aging, and discover what happens as we age:
- Cellular Senescence
- Telomere Shortening
- Epigenetic Changes
- Hormonal Shifts
- Mitochondrial Dysfunction

Let's dive deeper into each of these biological changes and their impact on our lives:

Cellular Senescence

As we age, our cells' ability to divide and grow slows down, leading to:

- Wrinkles and age spots due to reduced collagen production and skin elasticity
- Decreased energy levels and fatigue
- Increased risk of age-related diseases like cancer and atherosclerosis

Telomere Shortening

The protective caps on our chromosomes wear off, causing:

- Genetic damage and increased risk of disease
- Cellular aging and reduced cellular function
- Increased risk of cancer and age-related diseases

Epigenetic Changes

Our genes' expression is altered, influencing:

- Metabolism, leading to weight gain or loss, and increased risk of age-related diseases
- Inflammation, contributing to chronic diseases like arthritis and cardiovascular disease
- Cellular stress, leading to fatigue and decreased vitality

Hormonal Shifts

Our hormone levels fluctuate, impacting:

- Mood, leading to increased risk of depression and anxiety
- Energy levels, causing fatigue and decreased motivation
- Overall well-being, affecting sleep, appetite, and cognitive function

Mitochondrial Dysfunction

Our cells' energy-producing powerhouses decline, leading to:

- Fatigue and decreased vitality
- Increased risk of age-related diseases like Alzheimer's and Parkinson's
- Reduced physical performance and endurance

Our exploration of the biology of aging has revealed the complex and interconnected changes that occur in our bodies as we age. From cellular senescence to mitochondrial dysfunction, these changes can have a profound impact on our daily lives, relationships, and overall well-being. By understanding these changes, we can better appreciate the importance of promoting healthy aging and reducing the risk of age-related diseases."

CHAPTER 2: Impact of Lifestyle Choices on Aging

Meet Mark, a successful entrepreneur in his late 50s, who seemed to have it all - wealth, status, and a thriving business. However, his fast-paced lifestyle took a toll on his health. He was overweight, stressed, and struggling to keep up with the demands of his company.

One day, Mark's doctor delivered a wake-up call: "Your lifestyle is aging you faster than your years." Mark realized that his choices were not only affecting his health but also accelerating his aging process.

Let's explore how Mark's lifestyle choices impacted his aging process:

Nutrition

Mark's diet led to:

- Chronic inflammation, causing cellular damage and aging
- Increased risk of age-related diseases like diabetes, cardiovascular disease, and certain cancers
- Reduced energy levels and decreased vitality

Exercise

His sedentary lifestyle resulted in:

- Muscle loss and decreased mobility, affecting daily functioning and independence
- Reduced telomere length, accelerating cellular aging
- Increased risk of age-related diseases like osteoporosis and cognitive decline

Stress

Chronic stress caused:

- Epigenetic changes, influencing gene expression and aging
- Hormonal imbalances, affecting mood, energy, and overall well-being
- Mitochondrial dysfunction, reducing cellular energy production

Sleep

Poor sleep habits disrupted:

- Circadian rhythms, affecting cellular regeneration and immune function
- Cellular regeneration, leading to premature aging and increased disease risk
- Overall well-being, causing fatigue, mood disturbances, and decreased quality of life

Social Connections

Mark's lack of nurturing relationships led to:

- Feelings of loneliness and isolation, affecting mental health and well-being
- Reduced social support, increasing stress and decreasing resilience
- Negative impact on cognitive function and overall health

Through Mark's story, we see how lifestyle choices can accelerate aging. However, by making informed choices, we can decelerate the aging process, increase vitality, and reduce the risk of age-related diseases.

CHAPTER 3: Debunking Aging Myths: Separating Fact from Fiction

Meet Sophia, a vibrant and curious woman in her 60s, who was determined to separate fact from fiction when it came to aging. She had heard countless myths and misconceptions about growing older, and she wanted to know the truth.

Let's dive deeper into debunking these common aging myths with Sophia:

Myth 1: Aging means decline

Fact: Lifestyle choices like exercise, nutrition, and stress management can influence aging's impact.

Research: Studies show that regular exercise can improve physical function and reduce decline.

Expert insight: "Aging is not just about decline, but also about growth and transformation." - Dr. Laura Carstensen, Stanford Center on Longevity

Myth 2: Memory loss is inevitable

Fact: Brain exercises, social engagement, and cognitive training can help prevent memory loss.

Research: Cognitive training programs have shown to improve memory and cognitive function.

Expert insight: "The brain is capable of reorganizing itself throughout life." - Dr. Michael Merzenich, Neuroscientist

Myth 3: Older adults can't learn new things

Fact: Neuroplasticity allows our brains to adapt and learn throughout life.

Research: Studies show that older adults can learn new skills and languages.

Expert insight: "Age is not a barrier to learning."
- Dr. Barbara Strauch, Neuroscientist

Myth 4: Aging means losing your sense of purpose

Fact: Purpose can be rediscovered and reignited through new passions, relationships, and contributions.

Research: Studies show that having a sense of purpose can improve mental and physical health.

Expert insight: "Purpose is not something you find, it's something you create." - Dr. Richard Leider, Purpose Expert

Myth 5: Older adults are too old for technology

Fact: Technology can enhance life, and many older adults are embracing it.

Research: Studies show that technology can improve social connections and cognitive function.

Expert insight: "Technology can be a powerful tool for healthy aging." - Dr. Joseph Coughlin, MIT AgeLab

By exploring the latest research and expert insights, Sophia is discovering that aging is not just about decline, but also about growth, transformation, and new possibilities.

PART TWO: NUTRITION FOR LONGEVITY

CHAPTER 4: The Power of Nutrition: Fueling Your Body for Longevity

Meet Emma, a vibrant and energetic woman in her 40s, who was determined to take control of her health. She had heard the phrase "you are what you eat," but she never realized the profound impact of nutrition on her body's longevity.

Emma's journey began with a simple question: "What foods can help me live a longer, healthier life?" She discovered that nutrition is not just about sustenance, but about fueling her body for optimal performance.

Anti-Aging Foods

Emma learned about foods rich in antioxidants (berries, leafy greens), omega-3 fatty acids (salmon, walnuts), and fiber (legumes, whole grains) that combat inflammation and cellular damage.

Research: Studies show that antioxidants reduce oxidative stress, while omega-3 fatty acids support heart health.

Expert insight: "Food is the best medicine for aging." - Dr. David Sinclair, Harvard Geneticist

The Longevity Diet

Emma discovered the importance of whole, plant-based foods (fruits, vegetables, whole grains) for promoting cellular health and telomere length.

Research: Studies show that plant-based diets reduce chronic disease risk and promote longevity.

Expert insight: "Plant-based diets are the key to longevity." - Dr. Valter Longo, USC Longevity Institute

Nutrient-Dense Foods

Emma found out how foods like leafy greens (spinach, kale), berries (blueberries, strawberries), and nuts (walnuts, almonds) support mitochondrial function, energy production, and overall well-being.

Research: Studies show that these foods improve cognitive function, heart health, and immune response.

Expert insight: "Nutrient-dense foods are essential for optimal health." - Dr. Rhonda Patrick, FoundMyFitness

The Gut-Brain Connection

Emma learned how gut health impacts cognitive function, mood, and immune response, and how nutrition can support a healthy gut microbiome.

Research: Studies show that gut health is linked to brain health and immune function.

Expert insight: "The gut is the second brain." - Dr. Emeran Mayer, UCLA Gut-Brain Research

Personalized Nutrition

Emma realized that everyone's nutritional needs are unique and how genetic testing, biomarkers, and personalized coaching can help tailor her diet for optimal results.

Research: Studies show that personalized nutrition improves health outcomes and reduces disease risk.

Expert insight: "Personalized nutrition is the future of healthcare." - Dr. Robert Green, Harvard Geneticist

Through Emma's journey, we've explored the latest research and expert insights on the power of nutrition for longevity. We've discovered how food can be medicine, and how making informed choices can lead to a longer, healthier, and more vibrant life.

By incorporating anti-aging foods, following the longevity diet, eating nutrient-dense foods, supporting gut health, and personalizing her nutrition, Emma has taken control of her health and well-being. Her story serves as a reminder that nutrition is a powerful tool for promoting longevity and living a healthy, fulfilling life.

CHAPTER 5: The Top Foods for a Younger, Healthier You

Meet Olivia, a busy professional in her 30s, who wanted to regain her youthful energy and glow. She discovered that incorporating specific foods into her diet could help her achieve her goal.

Let's join Olivia on her journey to uncover the top foods for a younger, healthier her:

Leafy Greens: Olivia learned how spinach, kale, and collard greens support cellular health, reduce inflammation, and promote telomere length.

Berries: She discovered the antioxidant power of blueberries, raspberries, and strawberries in combating aging and oxidative stress.

Fatty Fish: Olivia found out how salmon, tuna, and sardines support heart health, reduce inflammation, and promote brain function.

Sweet Potatoes: She learned how this complex carbohydrate supports healthy digestion, immune function, and skin health.

Avocados: Olivia discovered the benefits of healthy fats in avocados for heart health, weight management, and glowing skin.

Legumes: She found out how beans, lentils, and chickpeas support healthy blood sugar, weight management, and cellular health.

Nuts and Seeds: Olivia learned about the antioxidant power of walnuts, chia seeds, and flaxseeds in supporting heart health and cognitive function.

Fermented Foods: She discovered the benefits of kimchi, sauerkraut, and kefir in supporting gut health and immune function.

Through Olivia's journey, we've uncovered the top foods for a younger, healthier her. These nutrient-dense foods have been shown to:

- Support cellular health and telomere length
- Reduce inflammation and oxidative stress
- Promote heart health and brain function
- Support healthy digestion, immune function, and skin health
- Provide healthy fats for weight management and glowing skin
- Support healthy blood sugar and cellular health
- Provide antioxidant power for heart health and cognitive function
- Support gut health and immune function

By incorporating these foods into her diet, Olivia has experienced:

- Increased energy levels
- Glowing, healthy skin
- Improved overall health and well-being
- A reduced risk of chronic diseases
- A stronger immune system

- Improved cognitive function and focus
- A more vibrant and youthful life

Through Olivia's story, we've seen the power of nutrition in achieving a younger, healthier self. By making informed food choices, we can take control of our health and well-being, and live a more vibrant, energetic life.

CHAPTER 6: Supplements and Nutrients for Optimal Health

Meet Alex, a fitness enthusiast in his 40s, who wanted to optimize his health and performance. He discovered that incorporating specific supplements and nutrients into his diet could help him achieve his goal.

Let's join Alex on his journey to uncover the top supplements and nutrients for optimal health:

Omega-3 Fatty Acids: Alex learned how fish oil supplements support heart health, reduce inflammation, and promote brain function.

Probiotics: He discovered the benefits of probiotics in supporting gut health, immune function, and digestion.

Vitamin D: Alex found out how vitamin D supplements support bone health, immune function, and mood regulation.

Coenzyme Q10 (CoQ10): He learned about the antioxidant power of CoQ10 in supporting energy production, heart health, and cellular function.

Turmeric/Curcumin: Alex discovered the anti-inflammatory benefits of curcumin in supporting joint health, cognitive function, and immune response.

Magnesium: He found out how magnesium supplements support muscle function, heart health, and stress relief.

Ashwagandha: Alex learned about the adaptogenic benefits of ashwagandha in supporting stress resilience, energy, and sleep quality.

Vitamin B Complex: He discovered the importance of B vitamins in supporting energy production, nerve function, and heart health.

Through Alex's journey, we've uncovered the top supplements and nutrients for optimal health. These essential nutrients have been shown to:

- Support heart health and reduce inflammation (Omega-3 Fatty Acids)
- Promote gut health, immune function, and digestion (Probiotics)
- Support bone health, immune function, and mood regulation (Vitamin D)
- Enhance energy production, heart health, and cellular function (Coenzyme Q10)
- Reduce inflammation and support joint health, cognitive function, and immune response (Turmeric/Curcumin)
- Support muscle function, heart health, and stress relief (Magnesium)
- Enhance stress resilience, energy, and sleep quality (Ashwagandha)
- Support energy production, nerve function, and heart health (Vitamin B Complex)

By incorporating these supplements into his diet, Alex has experienced:

- Increased energy levels and enhanced performance
- Improved heart health and reduced inflammation
- Stronger immune function and digestive health
- Enhanced cognitive function and mood regulation
- Improved joint health and reduced pain
- Better stress resilience and sleep quality
- Overall vibrant health and well-being

Remember to consult with a healthcare professional before adding any supplements to your diet. Through Alex's story, we've seen the potential benefits of incorporating these top supplements and nutrients into our lives. By making informed choices, we can take control of our health and optimize our well-being.

PART THREE: FITNESS AND EXERCISE

CHAPTER 7: The Importance of Exercise for Longevity

Meet Jack, a retired accountant in his 60s, who thought he was too old to start exercising. But after a wake-up call from his doctor, Jack discovered the transformative power of physical activity.

Let's join Jack on his journey to uncover the importance of exercise for longevity:

Cardiovascular Health: Jack learned how regular exercise strengthens his heart, lowers blood pressure, and improves circulation.

Muscle Mass and Strength: He discovered how resistance training builds muscle, boosts metabolism, and enhances bone density.

Cognitive Function: Jack found out how exercise improves memory, concentration, and cognitive processing speed.

Telomere Length: He learned about the link between exercise and longer telomeres, a key indicator of cellular aging.

Stress Reduction: Jack experienced firsthand how exercise reduces stress, anxiety, and depression.

Social Benefits: He discovered the joy of exercising with friends, building connections, and a sense of community.

Increased Energy: Jack found himself with more energy, vitality, and a zest for life.

Through Jack's journey, we've uncovered the numerous benefits of regular exercise for longevity. Exercise has been shown to:

- Strengthen cardiovascular health, lowering blood pressure and improving circulation
- Build muscle mass and strength, boosting metabolism and enhancing bone density
- Improve cognitive function, including memory, concentration, and processing speed
- Support telomere length, a key indicator of cellular aging
- Reduce stress, anxiety, and depression
- Foster social connections and a sense of community
- Increase energy levels, vitality, and overall zest for life

By incorporating regular exercise into his lifestyle, Jack has experienced:

- Improved overall health and well-being
- Enhanced physical function and mobility
- Better mental clarity and focus

- Reduced risk of chronic diseases
- Increased confidence and self-esteem
- A more vibrant and fulfilling life

Remember, exercise is a powerful tool for promoting longevity and overall health. By making physical activity a priority, we can take control of our health and well-being, and live a longer, healthier, and more vibrant life.

CHAPTER 8: Creating a Fitness Plan for a Younger, Healthier You

Meet Maya, a busy entrepreneur in her 30s, who wanted to regain her youthful energy and vitality. She discovered that creating a personalized fitness plan was the key to unlocking a younger, healthier her.

Let's join Maya on her journey to create a fitness plan that works:

Setting Goals: Maya learned how to set specific, achievable goals, such as increasing energy levels and improving overall health.

Assessing Fitness Levels: She discovered how to assess her current fitness level, including cardiovascular health, strength, and flexibility.

Choosing Activities: Maya found out how to select exercises she enjoys, such as swimming, cycling, and yoga, to make fitness a sustainable habit.

Creating a Schedule: She learned how to prioritize fitness and schedule workouts into her busy life.

Progress Tracking: Maya discovered the importance of tracking progress, celebrating milestones, and making necessary adjustments.

Mind-Body Connection: She experienced the transformative power of mind-body exercises, such as meditation and deep breathing, in reducing stress and increasing well-being.

Nutrition and Recovery: Maya learned how to fuel her body with a balanced diet and prioritize recovery techniques, such as stretching and foam rolling, for optimal results.

Through Maya's journey, we've uncovered the key elements of a personalized fitness plan. By:

- Setting specific, achievable goals
- Assessing her current fitness level
- Choosing enjoyable exercises
- Creating a schedule that prioritizes fitness
- Tracking progress and celebrating milestones
- Incorporating mind-body exercises for stress reduction and well-being
- Fueling her body with a balanced diet and prioritizing recovery techniques

Maya has experienced:

- Increased energy levels and vitality
- Improved overall health and well-being
- Enhanced physical function and mobility
- Reduced stress and anxiety
- Improved mental clarity and focus
- A more balanced and sustainable approach to fitness
- A younger, healthier, and more vibrant life

Remember, a personalized fitness plan is key to achieving success and maintaining motivation. By incorporating these elements, you can create a fitness plan that works for you and helps you reach your goals.

CHAPTER 9: Mind-Body Connection: The Role of Stress and Relaxation

Meet Sarah, a high-powered executive in her 40s, who thought she was thriving until she hit a wall of burnout. She discovered that her mind and body were intimately connected and that stress was sabotaging her well-being.

Let's join Sarah on her journey to uncover the mind-body connection:

The Stress Response: Sarah learned how chronic stress triggers a cascade of physiological reactions, impacting her mood, energy, and overall health.

The Relaxation Response: She discovered how relaxation techniques, such as deep breathing, meditation, and yoga, can calm her mind and body.

Mindfulness: Sarah found out how mindfulness practices, like journaling and walking, helped her stay present and focused.

Emotional Intelligence: She learned to recognize and manage her emotions, reducing stress and increasing resilience.

Gut-Brain Connection: Sarah discovered the fascinating link between her gut microbiome and brain function, and how nutrition impacts her mood and energy.

Sleep and Recovery: She prioritized sleep and recovery techniques, like progressive muscle relaxation and visualization, to rejuvenate her mind and body.

Through Sarah's journey, we've delved into the intricate relationships between stress, relaxation, mindfulness, emotional intelligence, gut-brain connection, and sleep. By understanding and addressing these aspects, Sarah has experienced:

- Reduced chronic stress and anxiety
- Improved mood and emotional regulation
- Enhanced focus, creativity, and productivity
- Better sleep quality and duration
- Increased energy and vitality
- Stronger resilience and adaptability
- Improved overall well-being and life satisfaction

By joining Sarah on this journey, we've discovered the transformative power of the mind-body connection. By managing stress, cultivating relaxation, and nurturing our mind-body relationship, we can unlock our full potential, leading to a more vibrant, creative, and fulfilling life.

Remember, the mind-body connection is a powerful tool for personal growth and transformation. By exploring and understanding this connection, we can take control of our well-being and live a more intentional, meaningful life.

PART FOUR: MIND AND SPIRIT

CHAPTER 10: The Power of Mindset: How Your Thoughts Impact Aging

Meet Maria, a vibrant woman in her 50s, who defied age expectations with her youthful energy and radiant glow. Her secret? A mindset shift that transformed her life.

Let's join Maria on her journey to uncover the power of mindset:

The Aging Mindset: Maria learned how societal expectations and negative self-talk can accelerate aging.

Reframing Thoughts: She discovered how to rewire her brain with positive affirmations, focusing on ability, not age.

Gratitude Practice: Maria found out how gratitude journaling and meditation cultivated a youthful outlook.

Purpose and Passion: She reignited her passions, discovering new purpose and drive.

Resilience: Maria learned to reframe challenges as opportunities, building resilience and confidence.

Mindful Aging: She embraced aging as a natural process, focusing on wisdom, experience, and growth.

Through Maria's journey, we've uncovered the profound impact of mindset on aging. By:

- Recognizing and challenging negative self-talk and societal expectations

- Reframing thoughts with positive affirmations and focusing on ability, not age
- Cultivating gratitude and a youthful outlook through journaling and meditation
- Reigniting passions and discovering new purpose and drive
- Building resilience and confidence by reframing challenges as opportunities
- Embracing aging as a natural process, focusing on wisdom, experience, and growth

Maria has experienced:

- Increased vitality and energy
- Enhanced creativity and inspiration
- Improved overall well-being and life satisfaction
- Stronger resilience and adaptability
- A more positive and empowered attitude towards aging
- A more fulfilling and purpose-driven life

By joining Maria on this journey, we've discovered the transformative power of mindset in aging. By harnessing the power of positive thinking, we can reverse negative aging patterns, cultivate vitality, and live a more intentional, meaningful life. Remember, thoughts have the power to shape our reality – choose to age with purpose, passion, and positivity!

CHAPTER 11: Secret Garden of Purpose: Cultivating Meaning for a Younger, Happier Life

Meet Emma, a successful businesswoman in her 30s, who felt unfulfilled and restless, despite her outward success. She embarked on a journey to discover her purpose and cultivate meaning, transforming her life forever.

Let's join Emma on her path to purpose:

The Purpose Paradox: Emma learned how societal expectations and pressure to conform can lead to a sense of emptiness.

Discovering Values: She uncovered her core values, passions, and strengths, and how they aligned with her purpose.

Exploring Interests: Emma experimented with new activities, reigniting old hobbies and discovering fresh ones.

Meaningful Connections: She nurtured relationships that supported her growth and purpose.

Purposeful Work: Emma transitioned to a career that aligned with her values, bringing fulfillment and joy.

Mindful Moments: She incorporated mindfulness practices, savoring life's beauty and wonder.

Living a purpose-driven life can lea,
d to increased happiness, vitality, and a more youthful spirit.

CHAPTER 12: Power of Connection: How Social Bonds Can Add Years to Your Life

Meet Rachel, a vibrant woman in her 60s, who credited her close-knit community for her youthful energy and longevity. Her story highlights the vital role of social connections in living a longer, happier life.

Let's join Rachel on her journey to discover the importance of social connections:

The Loneliness Epidemic: Rachel learned how isolation can lead to premature aging and increased mortality rates.

Building Bridges: She discovered the joy of nurturing relationships with family, friends, and neighbors.

Community Engagement: Rachel found purpose in volunteering, and connecting with like-minded individuals.

Social Support Network: She built a safety net of supportive people, reducing stress and anxiety.

Laughter and Play: Rachel prioritized fun, playful activities with friends, boosting her mood and immune system.

Intergenerational Connections: She fostered meaningful relationships with younger generations, staying vibrant and engaged.

Investing in relationships can lead to increased happiness, resilience, and a longer, healthier life.

PART FIVE: ADVANCED STRATEGIES

CHAPTER 13: Unlocking the Fountain of Youth: Cutting-Edge Therapies for Longevity

Meet Dr. Lee, a pioneering researcher in the field of longevity, who dedicated her life to uncovering innovative therapies to extend the human lifespan. Her story takes us on a journey to the forefront of cutting-edge treatments.

Let's join Dr. Lee on her quest to discover:

Senolytic Therapy: A revolutionary approach to removing senescent cells, reversing age-related diseases.

Stem Cell Therapy: Harnessing the power of stem cells to regenerate tissues, and restore vitality.

Gene Editing: The groundbreaking potential of CRISPR technology to rewrite genetic code, and prevent age-related diseases.

Mitochondrial Function: Unlocking the secrets of cellular energy, boosting longevity.

Personalized Medicine: Tailoring treatments to individual genetic profiles, optimizing results.

Mind-Body Therapies: Integrating meditation, yoga, and mindfulness to reduce stress, and promote well-being.

Dr. Lee's eyes sparkled as she gazed through the microscope, witnessing the miraculous transformation. Senescent cells, once thought to be irreversible, were vanishing before her eyes, thanks to the revolutionary senolytic therapy. This was just the beginning.

Next, she turned her attention to stem cell therapy, marveling at the ability of these tiny powerhouses to regenerate tissues and restore vitality. The potential was staggering – reversing age-related diseases, extending human lifespan, and improving healthspan.

But Dr. Lee didn't stop there. She delved into the groundbreaking world of gene editing, harnessing the power of CRISPR technology to rewrite genetic code and prevent age-related diseases. The possibilities were endless.

As she explored further, Dr. Lee became fascinated with mitochondrial function, unlocking the secrets of cellular energy and boosting longevity. She also discovered the importance of personalized medicine, tailoring treatments to individual genetic profiles for optimal results.

Finally, Dr. Lee turned her attention to mind-body therapies, integrating meditation, yoga, and mindfulness to reduce stress and promote well-being. The synergy was profound – a holistic approach to extending human lifespan, improving healthspan, and enhancing quality of life.

Dr. Lee's quest had uncovered a new frontier in human health and longevity. She was no longer just a scientist; she was a pioneer, blazing a trail towards a future where age-related diseases were a thing of the past.

CHAPTER 14: The Age-Proof Revolution: Emerging Trends and Technologies for a Younger Tomorrow

Meet Ava, a visionary entrepreneur, who embarked on a mission to harness the power of innovation to age-proof human life. Her story takes us on a fascinating journey to the forefront of emerging trends and technologies.

Let's join Ava on her quest to discover:

Personalized Aging Biomarkers: AI-driven diagnostics, identifying individual aging patterns, and predicting age-related diseases.

Regenerative Medicine: Groundbreaking therapies, harnessing stem cells, and bioactive molecules to revive tissues and organs.

Brain-Computer Interfaces: Revolutionary neurotechnologies, enhancing cognitive function, and unlocking human potential.

Age-Reversal Supplements: Cutting-edge nutrigenomics, and senolytic compounds, targeting cellular aging mechanisms.

Smart Homes for Healthy Aging: Innovative living spaces, integrating AI, and IoT, to support age-proof lifestyles.

Virtual Reality Age-Proofing: Immersive experiences, redefining mental and physical wellness, and cognitive function.

Ava's quest led her to the forefront of aging research, where she discovered personalized aging biomarkers that used AI-driven diagnostics to identify individual aging patterns and predict age-related diseases.

As she delved deeper, Ava explored regenerative medicine, uncovering groundbreaking therapies that harnessed stem cells and bioactive molecules to revive tissues and organs. She also encountered revolutionary brain-computer interfaces that enhanced cognitive function and unlocked human potential.

Ava's journey further took her to age-reversal supplements, cutting-edge nutrigenomics, and senolytic compounds that targeted cellular aging mechanisms. Additionally, she discovered smart homes designed for healthy aging, innovative living spaces that integrated AI and IoT to support age-proof lifestyles.

Finally, Ava ventured into virtual reality age-proofing, immersive experiences that redefined mental and physical wellness and cognitive function. Her quest had opened doors to a future where aging was no longer a limitation, but an opportunity to enhance and expand human life.

CHAPTER 15:Age-Proof Journey: Integrating Longevity into Everyday Life

Meet Sophia, a vibrant woman in her 50s, who embarked on a transformative journey to integrate age-proofing into her life. Her story takes us on a relatable and inspiring path to embracing longevity.

Let's join Sophia on her journey to discover:

Mindful Mornings: Starting each day with purpose, meditation, and movement to boost energy and clarity.

Nourishing Habits: Savoring whole foods, and embracing personalized nutrition for optimal well-being.

Movement Mastery: Incorporating age-defying exercises, like yoga and swimming, to strengthen body and mind.

Sleep Sanctuary: Crafting a restful sleep environment, and prioritizing restorative rest.

Social Connections: Cultivating meaningful relationships, and building a supportive community.

Continuous Learning: Embracing lifelong learning, and exploring new passions to stay curious and engaged.

Self-Care Rituals: Prioritizing stress-reducing activities, like reading and relaxation, to soothe the mind and body.

Sophia woke up to the gentle glow of dawn, signaling the start of her mindful morning routine. She began with meditation, focusing on her breath, and then transitioned to movement, her body flowing through yoga poses with grace and ease. This daily ritual set the tone for a purposeful day, filled with energy and clarity.

As she savored whole foods for breakfast, Sophia reflected on her nourishing habits, grateful for the personalized nutrition plan that optimized her well-being. Her day unfolded with movement mastery, incorporating age-defying exercises like swimming, strengthening both body and mind.

After a fulfilling day, Sophia retreated to her sleep sanctuary, a restful environment crafted to prioritize restorative rest. She knew that social connections were vital, too, and made time for meaningful relationships and community building.

Sophia's journey also emphasized continuous learning, embracing lifelong curiosity and exploring new passions. Her self-care rituals, like reading and relaxation, soothed her mind and body, reducing stress and promoting serenity.

Through these small yet profound changes, Sophia cultivated a vibrant, healthy, and fulfilling life – a testament to the power of intentional living.

CONCLUSION

Unlocking the Secrets of Longevity: A Summary of Key Takeaways

As we conclude our journey through the realms of age-proofing, let's reflect on the transformative insights and practical wisdom gathered along the way. Meet Rachel, a curious and adventurous individual, who embarked on a quest to distill the essence of longevity into actionable takeaways.

Join Rachel as she recounts the top key takeaways:

Embrace a Growth Mindset: Cultivate curiosity, resilience, and adaptability to thrive in an ever-changing world.

Nurture Mind-Body Connection: Prioritize self-care, stress reduction, and mindfulness to harmonize body and mind.

Fuel Your Body: Savor whole foods, and personalized nutrition, and stay hydrated for optimal energy and vitality.

Move with Purpose: Incorporate age-defying exercises, like yoga and swimming, to strengthen body and mind.

Cultivate Meaningful Connections: Build a supportive community, prioritize relationships, and stay socially engaged.

Stay Curious and Creative: Embrace lifelong learning, explore new passions, and nurture cognitive function.

Prioritize Sleep and Recovery: Craft a restful sleep environment, and prioritize restorative rest.

Harness Emerging Trends and Technologies:
Explore innovative therapies, AI-powered health analytics, and age-proofing technologies.

Rachel reflected on her journey, distilling the essence of her discoveries into eight vital keys. First, she emphasized the importance of embracing a growth mindset, cultivating curiosity, resilience, and adaptability to thrive in an ever-changing world.

Next, Rachel highlighted the need to nurture the mind-body connection, prioritizing self-care, stress reduction, and mindfulness to harmonize body and mind. She also stressed the importance of fueling her body with whole foods, personalized nutrition, and staying hydrated for optimal energy and vitality.

Rachel's fourth key was to move with purpose, incorporating age-defying exercises like yoga and swimming to strengthen body and mind. She also underscored the value of cultivating meaningful connections, building a supportive community, prioritizing relationships, and staying socially engaged.

The sixth key was to stay curious and creative, embracing lifelong learning, exploring new passions, and nurturing cognitive function. Rachel also emphasized the importance of prioritizing sleep and recovery, crafting a restful sleep environment, and prioritizing restorative rest.

Finally, Rachel encouraged harnessing emerging trends and technologies, exploring innovative therapies, AI-powered health analytics, and age-proofing technologies to stay ahead of the curve.

Through Rachel's story, we've recapped the essential insights and practical tips for embracing longevity with confidence and joy. By incorporating these eight keys, we can unlock the secrets of a vibrant, healthy, and fulfilling life.

The Age-Proof Odyssey: Embracing a Life of Vitality and Joy

Meet Alexandra, a vibrant and adventurous woman, who embarked on a transformative journey to embrace an age-proof lifestyle. Her story takes us on a captivating path of self-discovery, growth, and empowerment. Join Alexandra as she shares her inspiring journey:

Awakening to Age-Proofing: Discovering the power of mindset, self-care, and intentional living.

Nourishing Body and Soul: Embracing whole foods, personalized nutrition, and mindful eating.

Movement Mastery: Finding joy in age-defying exercises, like yoga, swimming, and dance.

Mindful Moments: Prioritizing stress reduction, meditation, and connection with nature.

Cultivating Connections: Building meaningful relationships, and staying socially engaged.

Continuous Growth: Embracing lifelong learning, exploring new passions, and nurturing creativity.

Resilience and Adaptability: Developing a growth mindset, and embracing life's challenges.

Age-Proofing with Intention: Integrating emerging trends, technologies, and innovative therapies.

The Age-Proof Journey: Final Thoughts and Next Steps

As we conclude our transformative journey through the realms of age-proofing, let's reflect on the profound insights and practical wisdom gathered along the way.

Maya is a wise and compassionate guide, who distills the essence of our odyssey into final thoughts and next steps.
Join Maya as she shares her heartfelt reflections:

Embrace Your Unique Journey: Celebrate individuality, and honor your distinct path.

Cultivate Mindfulness: Stay present, aware, and intentional in every moment.

Nurture Resilience: Develop a growth mindset, and embrace life's challenges.

Prioritize Connection: Foster meaningful relationships, and stay socially engaged.

Stay Curious: Embrace lifelong learning, and explore new passions.

Integrate Age-Proofing: Incorporate emerging trends, technologies, and innovative therapies.

Share Your Wisdom: Inspire others, and pay it forward.

Maya's final thoughts:

Age-proofing is a journey, not a destination. It's a mindset, a lifestyle, and a commitment to living your best life. Remember, every moment is an opportunity to grow, learn, and thrive.

Next steps:

Start small: Integrate one age-proofing practice into your daily life.

Seek community: Connect with like-minded individuals, and join the age-proofing movement.

Stay informed: Explore emerging trends, technologies, and innovative therapies.

Share your story: Inspire others, and pay it forward.

Maya smiled, knowing that age-proofing was a journey, not a destination. She had learned that it was a mindset, a lifestyle, and a commitment to living her best life. Every moment was an opportunity to grow, learn, and thrive.

As she looked to the future, Maya encouraged others to start small, integrating one age-proofing practice into their daily life. She knew the power of community and sought connections with like-minded individuals, joining the age-proofing movement.

Maya also emphasized the importance of staying informed, exploring emerging trends, technologies, and innovative therapies. And finally, she encouraged others to share their stories, inspiring others and paying it forward.

With these final thoughts, Maya's journey came full circle. She had discovered the secrets of age-proofing and was now ready to share them with the world. Join Maya and the age-proofing community in embracing a vibrant, healthy, and fulfilling life. Start your journey today!